Cortisol Reset for Women

A Step-by-Step 3-Week Plan to Manage Stress, Balance Hormones, and Reclaim Energy

copyright © 2025 Stephanie Hinderock

All rights reserved No part of this book may be reproduced, or stored in a retrieval system, or transmitted in any form or by any means, electronic, mechanical, photocopying, recording, or otherwise, without express written permission of the publisher.

Disclaimer

By reading this disclaimer, you are accepting the terms of the disclaimer in full. If you disagree with this disclaimer, please do not read the guide.

All of the content within this guide is provided for informational and educational purposes only, and should not be accepted as independent medical or other professional advice. The author is not a doctor, physician, nurse, mental health provider, or registered nutritionist/dietician. Therefore, using and reading this guide does not establish any form of a physician-patient relationship.

Always consult with a physician or another qualified health provider with any issues or questions you might have regarding any sort of medical condition. Do not ever disregard any qualified professional medical advice or delay seeking that advice because of anything you have read in this guide. The information in this guide is not intended to be any sort of medical advice and should not be used in lieu of any medical advice by a licensed and qualified medical professional.

The information in this guide has been compiled from a variety of known sources. However, the author cannot attest to or guarantee the accuracy of each source and thus should not be held liable for any errors or omissions.

You acknowledge that the publisher of this guide will not be held liable for any loss or damage of any kind incurred as a result of this guide or the reliance on any information provided within this guide. You acknowledge and agree that you assume all risk and responsibility for any action you undertake in response to the information in this guide.

Using this guide does not guarantee any particular result (e.g., weight loss or a cure). By reading this guide, you acknowledge that there are no guarantees to any specific outcome or results you can expect.

All product names, diet plans, or names used in this guide are for identification purposes only and are the property of their respective owners. The use of these names does not imply endorsement. All other trademarks cited herein are the property of their respective owners.

Where applicable, this guide is not intended to be a substitute for the original work of this diet plan and is, at most, a supplement to the original work for this diet plan and never a direct substitute. This guide is a personal expression of the facts of that diet plan.

Where applicable, persons shown in the cover images are stock photography models and the publisher has obtained the rights to use the images through license agreements with third-party stock image companies.

Table of Contents

Introduction	**8**
Understanding Cortisol & Women's Health	**10**
What Is Cortisol?	10
How Cortisol Impacts Female Hormones	11
Signs of Cortisol Imbalance in Women	13
Myths About Stress and Cortisol	15
The Science Behind the Cortisol Reset	**18**
Chronic Stress and the HPA Axis	18
Cortisol, Weight Gain, and Belly Fat	19
Cortisol and Sleep Disruption	20
Why Women Are More Affected by Cortisol Dysregulation	20
Getting Ready: Reset Mindset & Daily Prep	**22**
Setting Realistic Goals	22
Creating a Supportive Routine	23
Pantry Detox and Grocery Essentials	24
Journaling and Self-Awareness Practices	27
Foods That Heal, Foods That Harm	**29**
Anti-Inflammatory Foods for Cortisol Balance	29
What to Avoid: Stimulants, Sugar, and Processed Carbs	31
The Role of Protein, Fats, and Adaptogens	33
Sample Shopping List	35
The 3-Week Cortisol Reset Plan	**38**
Week 1: Calm the Body	38
Week 2: Nourish & Repair (Days 8–14)	46
Week 3: Sustain & Strengthen (Days 15–21)	50
Daily Rituals for Stress Support	54
Meal Plans & Recipes	**57**
7-Day Sample Meal Plan	57
Cortisol-Balancing Breakfasts	61

Overnight Chia Oats	62
Veggie Breakfast Scramble	63
Protein-Packed Smoothie Bowl	64
Energy-Stabilizing Lunches	65
Quinoa Salad with Roasted Vegetables	66
Lentil and Arugula Salad	67
Mediterranean Veggie Wrap	68
Hormone-Supportive Dinners	69
Salmon and Broccoli Dinner	69
Chicken Stir-Fry with Veggies	70
Turmeric Cod with Sweet Potatoes	71
Calming Teas, Snacks & Smoothies	**72**
Calming Teas	73
Chamomile Lavender Tea	73
Ginger-Turmeric Tea	74
Holy Basil (Tulsi) Tea	75
Nutrient-Dense Snacks	76
Coconut Chia Seed Energy Bites	76
Roasted Chickpeas with Spices	77
Sliced Veggies with Avocado Dip	78
Relaxing Smoothies	79
Blueberry-Banana Calm Smoothie	79
Ashwagandha Adaptogen Smoothie	80
Chocolate Almond Bliss Smoothie	81
Lifestyle Habits That Reset Cortisol	**82**
Gentle Movement & Walking Protocols	82
Sleep Optimization	84
Breathing Exercises & Grounding Techniques	85
Reducing Screen Time and Cortisol Triggers	88
Beyond the Reset: Long-Term Stress Management	**90**
How to Reintroduce Foods Without Relapse	90

Building Resilience: Mental & Physical	92
Monitoring Progress and Listening to Your Body	94
When to Seek Help: Doctors, Labs, & Next Steps	95
Conclusion	**98**
FAQs	**100**
References and Helpful Links	**103**

Introduction

Stress has a way of creeping into daily life, affecting both body and mind in ways that often go unnoticed until it's too late. For women, the stakes are even higher, as fluctuating hormones and packed schedules can make it harder to maintain balance. At the heart of it all lies cortisol, the body's primary stress hormone. While it plays an essential role in managing energy, metabolism, and the fight-or-flight response, an overproduction of cortisol can wreak havoc on health, leading to fatigue, weight gain, mood swings, and even hormonal imbalances.

Navigating through constant demands, both personal and professional, only adds to the challenge. Modern life is full of triggers that send cortisol levels soaring, from hurried mornings to late nights spent scrolling through phones. Yet, finding calm amid the chaos isn't just a luxury; it's essential for long-term well-being. Managing cortisol is not about eliminating stress altogether but about building better habits that promote resilience and equilibrium.

In this guide, we will talk about the following:

- Understanding Cortisol & Women's Health
- The Science Behind the Cortisol Reset
- Anti-Inflammatory Foods for Cortisol Balance
- The 3-Week Cortisol Reset Plan
- Meal Plans & Recipes
- Lifestyle Habits That Reset Cortisol
- Beyond the Reset: Long-Term Stress Management

Keep reading to learn more about cortisol and how you can take control of your stress levels for better overall health and well-being. By the end of this guide, you will have a better understanding of cortisol and how it affects your body, as well as strategies for managing and balancing your levels to improve your overall quality of life.

Understanding Cortisol & Women's Health

Understanding the role of cortisol, also known as the "stress hormone", in women's health is crucial for maintaining overall well-being. In this chapter, we will explore the basics of cortisol and its impact on women's bodies.

What Is Cortisol?

Cortisol, commonly known as the "stress hormone," is a crucial hormone produced by the adrenal glands located just above your kidneys. Despite its negative reputation, cortisol serves many essential functions in the body. It acts as your built-in alarm system, kicking into action whenever a threat is detected.

By releasing glucose into your bloodstream, it provides the energy needed for a quick "fight or flight" response, enhances focus, increases heart rate, and temporarily slows down non-essential processes like digestion and growth.

But cortisol isn't just about stress. It's crucial for everyday functions like regulating metabolism, supporting your immune system, maintaining your blood pressure, and ensuring you have enough energy to get through the day. For example, cortisol helps wake you up in the morning and keeps your body active and alert throughout the day. Ideally, cortisol should rise in the morning, decrease gradually by the afternoon, and remain low at night, allowing you to sleep peacefully.

When stress becomes chronic, however, cortisol production can go haywire. Your body may produce too much or too little, which throws off balance in many systems. For women, this imbalance can uniquely affect reproductive health, energy levels, and emotional well-being.

How Cortisol Impacts Female Hormones

Hormonal balance is delicate, especially for women. Cortisol doesn't act in isolation; it interacts with other hormones like estrogen, progesterone, and testosterone. When cortisol levels stay elevated for long periods, it can disrupt this balance and significantly impact your overall health.

The "Pregnenolone Steal"

Your body produces cortisol from a hormone called pregnenolone, which is also used to produce progesterone. When stress is high and your body prioritizes cortisol production, it leaves less pregnenolone available to make other hormones.

This phenomenon, often referred to as the "pregnenolone steal," can cause a drop in progesterone levels. Why does this matter? Low progesterone can lead to symptoms like irregular periods, worsened PMS, and difficulty maintaining pregnancy, which is why stress and fertility are so closely linked.

The Impact on Estrogen Levels

Chronic stress can also disrupt estrogen levels, either raising or lowering them in a way that creates havoc for your menstrual cycle. High cortisol can signal your body to break down estrogen more quickly, leaving you with symptoms like heavy or irregular periods, mood swings, and even worsened menopausal symptoms.

Links to PCOS

For women with Polycystic Ovary Syndrome (PCOS) or other hormonal disorders, cortisol imbalances can worsen symptoms like weight gain, acne, and insulin resistance. Since cortisol affects blood sugar regulation, frequent stress can increase cravings for sugary, high-carb foods, leading to more unstable blood sugar levels and further hormonal disruption.

Fertility and Stress

Chronic stress, and by extension high cortisol, can interfere with ovulation. When your body feels "under attack," it prioritizes functions necessary for survival, not reproduction. Over time, this can lead to difficulty conceiving, even in women who were previously fertile.

All of these interconnected effects highlight just how critical cortisol is for women's hormonal health. Managing stress isn't just about feeling good emotionally; it's necessary for maintaining your physical health, menstrual cycles, and overall well-being.

Signs of Cortisol Imbalance in Women

What does cortisol imbalance look like in day-to-day life? Symptoms can vary widely, but there are some common signals to watch for. These symptoms often build up over time, making it easy to dismiss them as "just being tired" or "just being stressed." The truth is, these are your body's way of telling you it's overwhelmed.

1. **Chronic Fatigue**

    One of the most common signs of cortisol imbalance is feeling perpetually tired. Maybe you struggle to get out of bed in the morning (a sign your cortisol isn't rising properly), or maybe you experience a major energy slump mid-afternoon. Either way, despite feeling tired, you might also have trouble falling asleep or staying asleep at night, as cortisol peaks at the wrong times of day.

2. **Weight Gain, Especially Around the Belly**

   Cortisol directly influences where and how your body stores fat. When levels are high, your body tends to store fat in the abdominal region. This is not just a cosmetic issue—increased belly fat (also known as visceral fat) is linked to higher risks of heart disease and type 2 diabetes. You may also find it harder to lose weight, even with a healthy diet and exercise, because cortisol can slow your metabolism.

3. **Cravings for Sugar or Salt**

   Do you find yourself reaching for salty chips or sugary treats when you're stressed? This is another telltale sign of cortisol imbalance. High cortisol disrupts your blood sugar levels, leading to intense cravings for quick energy sources.

4. **Mood Swings and Anxiety**

   Unexplained irritability, heightened anxiety, or feeling emotionally "on edge" can signal cortisol dysregulation. High cortisol activates your body's fight-or-flight stress response, which, over time, can lead to increased sensitivity to emotional triggers.

5. **Hormonal Symptoms**

   Missed or irregular periods, worsened PMS, increased hair thinning, or even more severe menopausal symptoms can all point to underlying cortisol issues. If hormonal imbalances persist, they can impact every aspect of your health, from fertility to bone density.

6. **Digestive Issues**

   Cortisol slows down digestion during stress. If you're experiencing bloating, irregular bowel movements, or tummy troubles, unchecked stress might be the culprit.

Paying attention to these symptoms is crucial. Rather than accepting them as normal or unavoidable, you can take intentional steps to rebalance cortisol and help your body heal.

Myths About Stress and Cortisol

When it comes to cortisol and stress, misinformation abounds. It's easy to fall into myths that prevent you from addressing the real issue. Here are a few common misconceptions:

Myth #1: Stress Is Inevitable, and There's Nothing You Can Do About It

Many women feel resigned to chronic stress because they juggle so much—from careers to family obligations to societal expectations. While it's true that stress can't always be eliminated, it can be managed. You have more control over your stress response (and therefore your cortisol levels) than you might think. Strategies like mindfulness, proper nutrition, and setting boundaries can make a big difference. It starts with small, intentional changes.

Myth #2: Cortisol Is Always Bad

Cortisol often gets a bad rap, but it's not inherently "bad." It's a hormone your body needs to function properly. The problem arises when cortisol is either too high or too low. Keeping it in balance—not eliminating it entirely—is the goal. Remember, cortisol is what gives you energy in the morning and helps regulate important processes throughout your body.

Myth #3: You Just Need to "Relax More"

While relaxing activities like spa days and bubble baths can be helpful, managing cortisol requires a more comprehensive approach. Diet, sleep, exercise, and mental health practices all play significant roles in cortisol regulation. Effective stress management is about creating a holistic routine that nourishes your mind and body.

Myth #4: It's All in Your Head

If your symptoms aren't visible, some people might dismiss the idea of "cortisol issues" as overthinking. Rest assured, cortisol imbalances are real physiological changes that affect multiple systems in your body. These changes can be measured through lab tests and are backed by science.

Myth #5: Only Highly Stressed People Have Cortisol Problems

Even if you don't think of yourself as a "stressed-out" person, you may still struggle with cortisol regulation. Subtle but consistent stressors, like lack of sleep, dietary choices, or even over-exercising, can disrupt your cortisol levels over time.

By addressing these myths, you can move toward a healthier relationship with stress and better understanding of cortisol's role in your life.

Understanding how cortisol functions, its impact on women's hormonal health, and the signs of an imbalance is the first step. Armed with this knowledge, you can begin to take control of your well-being, empowering yourself to make changes that support your health and vitality. The chapters ahead will guide you through actionable steps to reset your cortisol levels and find sustainable relief from the effects of chronic stress.

The Science Behind the Cortisol Reset

Cortisol is sometimes called the "stress hormone," and for good reason. It plays a major role in how your body handles stress, energy, and even sleep. While cortisol is essential for survival, too much or too little can throw your body out of balance.

For women, this imbalance can lead to a host of issues, from disrupted sleep to stubborn belly fat. To reset your cortisol levels, it's important to first understand the science behind it. Let's break it down into simple, manageable pieces.

Chronic Stress and the HPA Axis

When you're stressed, your body activates something called the HPA axis, which stands for the hypothalamic-pituitary-adrenal axis. Think of it as your body's stress control system. Here's how it works:

- The brain (your hypothalamus) detects stress and signals your pituitary gland.

- The pituitary then tells your adrenal glands to release cortisol to help you handle the challenge.

Cortisol is helpful in small doses. It gives you energy, keeps you alert, and helps manage things like blood sugar and blood pressure. But chronic stress keeps the HPA axis turned on for too long, flooding your system with cortisol. This constant state of high stress wears down your body over time, affecting nearly every part of your well-being, especially for women who often juggle multiple responsibilities at once.

Cortisol, Weight Gain, and Belly Fat

One of cortisol's roles is to regulate blood sugar so you have energy during stressful moments. However, when cortisol remains high for long periods, your body stores more fat, especially around your belly. This is not just about aesthetics; abdominal fat is linked to a higher risk of heart disease and diabetes.

Why does this happen? Chronic stress often leads to sugar cravings. Eating sugary foods gives you a quick boost of energy, but it also causes blood sugar spikes. Cortisol then steps in to stabilize your blood sugar, but this cycle of stress eating and energy dips fuels further weight gain. Belly fat also produces its own hormones that can make cortisol regulation even harder. This is why managing cortisol isn't only about feeling good but also about protecting your long-term health.

Cortisol and Sleep Disruption

Cortisol plays a big role in how well you sleep and wake. Normally, cortisol levels peak in the morning to help you wake up and gradually drop throughout the day, hitting their lowest point at night when it's time to sleep.

If cortisol is too high, though, it disrupts this cycle. You may feel wired when you should be winding down, leading to insomnia or restless nights. On the flip side, constantly low cortisol can make it hard to feel alert in the morning, leaving you groggy and sluggish no matter how much sleep you've had.

Resetting cortisol begins with prioritizing good sleep hygiene. Sticking to a regular sleep schedule, limiting caffeine, and winding down with calming routines can help rebuild a healthy cortisol rhythm.

Why Women Are More Affected by Cortisol Dysregulation

Women's bodies are uniquely sensitive to cortisol changes for several reasons. Hormones like estrogen and progesterone interact with cortisol, meaning fluctuations during menstruation, pregnancy, or menopause can amplify stress responses. For instance:

- ***Estrogen***: High estrogen levels during certain times of the menstrual cycle can make cortisol more potent, intensifying its effects.
- ***Menopause***: During menopause, lower estrogen levels can disrupt cortisol balance, leading to more stress-related symptoms, like weight gain or insomnia.
- ***Societal pressures***: Women often face stress from juggling work, home, caregiving, and social expectations. This chronic stress can lead to persistent cortisol elevation.

What's particularly tricky is that high or prolonged cortisol can also impact other hormone systems, like thyroid hormones or insulin, which can add to women's struggles with fatigue, weight, and mood swings.

If cortisol is impacting your well-being, there are effective ways to reset and manage your levels. Strategies such as reducing stress, improving sleep habits, exercising in moderation, and maintaining a balanced diet can help restore cortisol balance and support your body's overall health.

Cortisol is a powerful hormone that responds to stress, but too much can cause major disruptions in your weight, sleep, and overall health. By making small, intentional changes, you can support your body's natural ability to find balance and feel your best again. And as women, it's more important than ever to give ourselves grace and prioritize self-care in this busy, demanding world.

Getting Ready: Reset Mindset & Daily Prep

Before beginning your cortisol reset, preparation is essential. Taking the time to set clear goals and create a supportive environment will improve your chances of success. This chapter focuses on the foundational steps needed to align your mindset, lifestyle, and surroundings for optimal results.

Setting Realistic Goals

Big changes don't happen overnight, and trying to do too much at once can set you up for frustration. That's why realistic, manageable goals are so crucial. They keep things achievable and help you celebrate small wins, which add up over time.

- ***Be specific***. Instead of saying, "I want to eat healthier," try, "I will eat one extra serving of vegetables every day." Small, clear goals give you direction and make it easier to stay consistent.
- ***Break it down***. Larger goals, like losing weight or lowering stress, can feel daunting. Break them into

smaller steps, like walking 20 minutes most days, practicing deep breathing, or cutting back on sugary drinks.
- *Track your progress*. Use a journal, app, or calendar to track your progress. Seeing how far you've come will motivate you to keep going.
- *Be kind to yourself*. Life happens, and no one is perfect. If you slip up, don't dwell on it. Acknowledge it, adjust, and move forward.

Setting realistic goals is key to creating lasting change without feeling overwhelmed. Focus on small, specific steps, track your progress, and remember to be patient with yourself along the way.

Creating a Supportive Routine

Women juggle a million things daily, so creating a routine that supports your goals is key. A solid routine helps reduce decision fatigue, so you don't have to think twice about healthy choices.

1. *Start with mornings*: A good day starts the night before. Set up your morning for success by prepping meals, laying out clothes, or planning a quick moment for yourself, like stretching or journaling. Even five minutes can make a difference.
2. *Be realistic with your time*: If you're already stretched thin, don't add an hour-long workout to your plate.

Instead, schedule something simple, like a 15-minute walk or a quick yoga session.
3. ***Prioritize consistency over perfection***: It's not about doing everything perfectly but doing it regularly. Even small, consistent habits, like drinking a glass of water first thing in the morning, help build momentum.
4. ***Identify your energy peaks***: Pay attention to when you feel most energized during the day and plan key tasks or workouts then. Protect those moments to focus on what matters most.

Your routine doesn't need to be rigid. It's okay to adapt as needed. The goal is to create structure while giving yourself room to breathe.

Pantry Detox and Grocery Essentials

Food plays a powerful role in resetting cortisol. While your body's stress response can't distinguish between emotional or physiological stress, the choices you make in the kitchen directly affect how your body responds. This step focuses on removing stress-inducing items from your pantry and restocking with nourishing options.

Foods that Hinder Cortisol Balance

Certain foods can lead to cortisol spikes or worsen hormonal disruptions:

- ***Refined sugars***: These cause rapid blood sugar fluctuations, triggering more cortisol production. Swap cakes, cookies, and sugary cereals for natural sweeteners like honey or maple syrup in moderation.
- ***Processed carbs***: White bread, crackers, and pasta offer little nutritional support and may spike blood sugar. Choose whole-grain alternatives instead.
- ***Caffeine***: While small amounts of coffee or tea can be fine, too much caffeine overstimulates the nervous system. Reduce intake gradually to avoid withdrawal symptoms.
- ***Alcohol***: Alcohol may feel relaxing in the moment, but it interferes with your sleep cycle and increases cortisol levels the next day.

Cortisol-Balancing Essentials

Stocking your kitchen with supportive foods makes it easier to maintain balance. Focus on these categories:

- ***Anti-inflammatory foods***: Leafy greens, berries, turmeric, ginger, and fatty fish like salmon can reduce inflammation, which is often elevated in those with high cortisol.
- ***Protein***: Lean meats, eggs, and plant-based options like quinoa and lentils help stabilize energy and blood sugar.

- *Healthy fats*: Avocados, nuts, seeds, and olive oil support brain health and help fuel your body without triggering blood sugar spikes.
- *Adaptogens*: Herbs like ashwagandha, holy basil, and maca root naturally support the body's stress response and promote cortisol regulation.

Sample Grocery List

Here's a list of essentials to get you started:

- Fresh produce like spinach, kale, zucchini, asparagus, apples, and blueberries.
- Healthy fat sources like almond butter, walnuts, chia seeds, and flaxseeds.
- Lean proteins such as chicken breast, turkey, eggs, and tofu.
- Herbal teas like chamomile, peppermint, and rooibos for calming evening rituals.
- Whole grains like quinoa, brown rice, and rolled oats.
- Adaptogenic supplements or teas (look for blends containing ashwagandha, reishi mushroom, or holy basil).

Detoxing your pantry may feel overwhelming initially, but taking it step by step makes the process manageable. Begin by replacing one processed item per week with a more nutritious alternative.

Journaling and Self-Awareness Practices

A successful cortisol reset isn't just about what you eat or how much you sleep; it's also about improving your relationship with stress. Journaling is a simple yet impactful way to uncover stress patterns and foster gratitude, self-reflection, and emotional resilience.

How Journaling Helps

Writing down your thoughts provides clarity and helps you process emotions. It encourages you to pause and focus on your inner world, interrupting the stress cycle. Journaling also allows you to track your progress, identify triggers, and recognize how small habits have a big impact on your well-being.

Daily Prompts to Get Started

If you're new to journaling, prompts can guide you:

- *Morning reflections*: "What are three things I'm grateful for today?"
- *Stress check-in*: "What felt stressful today, and how did I respond? What can I do differently next time?"
- *Goal review*: "What positive steps did I take toward my health goals this week?"
- *Gratitude practice*: "Write about one person, event, or moment that brought you joy today."

It's easy to feel discouraged if results aren't immediate, but journaling helps you see how far you've come. Use it to note improvements in your energy, mood, or sleep over time. You can even create a simple chart to record daily habits like taking walks, eating nutrient-dense meals, or practicing relaxation techniques.

Preparation is a crucial part of the cortisol reset process. By setting realistic goals, building supportive routines, detoxing your pantry, and cultivating self-awareness, you create a strong foundation for lasting change. These steps help shift your focus from stress to empowerment, giving you the tools to reclaim your health and well-being.

Foods That Heal, Foods That Harm

The food you eat doesn't just fuel your body; it has a direct impact on how your hormones function, including cortisol. By making intentional food choices, you can support your body's natural stress-management systems, reduce inflammation, and stabilize your energy. This chapter will help you understand which foods promote cortisol balance and which ones may be sabotaging your efforts.

Anti-Inflammatory Foods for Cortisol Balance

Inflammation is often described as the root cause of many chronic health issues, and high cortisol can both exacerbate and result from inflammation. Chronic, low-grade inflammation keeps your body in a heightened state of alert, triggering the stress response and making it harder to regulate cortisol levels. Incorporating anti-inflammatory foods into your diet can help calm this process.

Why Anti-Inflammatory Foods Matter

When inflammation is reduced, your body becomes better equipped to handle stress and maintain hormonal balance. These foods don't just assist with cortisol regulation; they also support your immune system, digestion, and overall energy levels.

Foods that Fight Inflammation

Here are some nutrient-rich options to prioritize in your meals:

- *Leafy Greens*: Spinach, kale, and arugula are packed with antioxidants and vitamins like vitamin C, which can lower stress hormone levels.
- *Colorful Veggies*: Think bell peppers, broccoli, carrots, and zucchini. These are full of phytonutrients that help combat oxidative stress.
- *Berries*: Blueberries, strawberries, and raspberries are loaded with antioxidants like anthocyanins, which reduce inflammation and support brain health.
- *Fatty Fish*: Salmon, mackerel, and sardines are rich in omega-3 fatty acids, known for their strong anti-inflammatory properties.
- *Nuts and Seeds*: Almonds, walnuts, chia seeds, and flaxseeds provide healthy fats and magnesium, a mineral that helps regulate stress.

- ***Herbs and Spices***: Incorporate turmeric, ginger, garlic, and cinnamon into your cooking for an anti-inflammatory boost.

Adding these foods to your meals doesn't have to be complicated. For example, a quick breakfast of oatmeal topped with chia seeds and berries or a salmon salad with avocado and leafy greens can deliver powerful anti-inflammatory benefits.

What to Avoid: Stimulants, Sugar, and Processed Carbs

While some foods help heal and balance your body, others can undermine your progress. Certain foods and substances increase cortisol levels by either spiking your blood sugar or overstimulating your nervous system. Removing (or at least reducing) these from your diet can make a significant difference in how you feel.

How These Foods Impact Cortisol

Stress-inducing foods contribute to cortisol imbalance by causing blood sugar swings, promoting inflammation, and putting unnecessary stress on your body's systems. Over time, this creates a vicious cycle of fatigue, cravings, and even more stress.

Culprits to Watch Out For

Here are some common foods and substances that may be throwing off your cortisol levels:

1. ***Refined Sugar***: Found in sodas, candies, pastries, and sweetened beverages, refined sugar triggers rapid blood sugar spikes, leading to a cortisol surge as your body struggles to stabilize.
    - <u>**Swap it with**</u>: Natural sweeteners like raw honey, maple syrup, or stevia (in moderation).
2. ***Processed Carbohydrates***: White bread, crackers, and chips are stripped of fiber and nutrients, causing a similar blood sugar crash-and-crave cycle.
    - <u>**Swap it with**</u>: Whole grains like quinoa, brown rice, and sprouted grain bread.
3. ***Caffeine***: While a morning cup of coffee is fine for many people, over-reliance on caffeine can overstimulate your adrenal glands, keeping cortisol levels elevated.
    - <u>**Swap it with**</u>: Herbal teas like chamomile, rooibos, or peppermint, or opt for a single cup of black tea if you need a caffeine boost.
4. ***Alcohol***: While it's tempting to unwind with a drink, alcohol increases cortisol production and disrupts your sleep cycles, making long-term stress management harder.

- **Swap it with**: Sparkling water with a splash of citrus or kombucha for a refreshing alternative.

Avoiding these foods might seem daunting at first, but simple substitutions can help you stay on track while still enjoying your meals.

The Role of Protein, Fats, and Adaptogens

A diet for cortisol balance isn't just about avoiding certain foods; it's also about ensuring you're eating enough of the right nutrients. Protein, healthy fats, and adaptogens all play vital roles in bringing cortisol levels back to baseline.

1. **Protein for Blood Sugar Stability**

    Protein is a key player in stabilizing blood sugar levels, which is essential for keeping cortisol under control. It also helps repair tissues and supports muscle recovery, which can take a hit when you're stressed.

    Good protein sources: Lean chicken, turkey, eggs, tofu, lentils, quinoa, and Greek yogurt.

    Aim to include a serving of protein in every meal, such as eggs for breakfast, a lentil soup for lunch, and grilled chicken with roasted veggies for dinner.

2. **Healthy Fats for Hormone Health**

   Far from being the enemy, healthy fats are essential for supporting brain function, reducing inflammation, and stabilizing hormones, including cortisol.

   Good fat sources: Avocados, nuts, seeds, olive oil, and fatty fish.

   For example, adding a tablespoon of chia seeds to your morning smoothie or drizzling olive oil over a salad can provide your body with the fats it needs to stay balanced.

3. **Adaptogens for Stress Support**

   Adaptogens are herbs and roots that help your body adapt to stress and normalize cortisol levels. Incorporating them into your diet can provide additional support for your adrenal system.

   <u>Popular adaptogens:</u>

   - *Ashwagandha*: Known for its ability to lower cortisol and promote relaxation.
   - *Holy Basil*: Helps improve focus and reduce stress-related symptoms.
   - *Reishi Mushroom*: Supports the immune system and aids sleep.

Adaptogens can be taken as capsules, added to smoothies, or consumed as teas. Start with one or two that suit your needs, and note how they impact your energy and stress levels.

Sample Shopping List

To help you put these principles into practice, here's a practical shopping list of foods and ingredients that support cortisol balance. Organize it by sections to make shopping easier:

Produce

- Leafy greens (spinach, kale, chard)
- Cruciferous vegetables (broccoli, cauliflower, Brussels sprouts)
- Berries (blueberries, raspberries, strawberries)
- Avocados
- Sweet potatoes

Proteins

- Wild-caught salmon
- Organic chicken or turkey
- Eggs
- Greek yogurt
- Lentils
- Quinoa

Healthy Fats

- Olive oil
- Coconut oil
- Walnuts
- Almonds
- Chia seeds
- Flaxseeds

Herbs and Spices

- Turmeric
- Ginger
- Cinnamon
- Garlic

Adaptogens

- Ashwagandha powder or capsules
- Holy basil (as tea or tincture)
- Reishi mushroom powder

Pantry Staples

- Herbal teas (chamomile, rooibos, peppermint)
- Bone broth
- Oats (steel-cut or rolled)
- Brown rice

By keeping your kitchen stocked with these items, you'll make it easier to prepare nourishing meals that work with your body, not against it.

Balancing your cortisol levels starts with what's on your plate. By focusing on anti-inflammatory, nutrient-dense foods and reducing inflammatory foods and stimulants, you give your body the building blocks it needs to heal. The next chapter will introduce a structured plan to incorporate these principles into your daily life for lasting results.

The 3-Week Cortisol Reset Plan

If you've been feeling stressed, worn out, or out of balance, resetting your cortisol levels may be just what you need to regain control of your well-being. This 3-week cortisol reset plan is designed to support your body and mind by addressing stress, nourishing your system, and building long-term resiliency. Follow the day-by-day guidance to ease into calming routines, repair your body, and strengthen habits that keep cortisol levels balanced.

Week 1: Calm the Body

Week 1 is all about setting the foundation for reducing stress and bringing both your body and mind into a calmer state. Through intentional activities, mindful habits, and small lifestyle adjustments, you'll begin to balance your nervous system and lower cortisol levels. This week prepares you for deeper healing in the weeks ahead, so each step you take is essential.

Days 1 & 2

1. ***Start with Breathwork***: Breathwork is a powerful way to reset your nervous system and lower cortisol levels almost instantly. Slow, intentional breathing signals your body to shift from "fight or flight" mode into a state of relaxation.

   Detailed Practice

   Find a comfortable spot in a quiet room to begin your breathing exercises. Sit with your back straight, shoulders relaxed, and feet flat on the ground. The 4-4-6 method is simple and effective:

   - *Step 1*: Breathe in deeply through your nose for 4 seconds.
   - *Step 2*: Hold your breath calmly for 4 seconds.
   - *Step 3*: Slowly exhale through your mouth for 6 seconds, feeling your chest and stomach decompress.

   Repeat this cycle 3–5 times, or for up to 10 minutes if you have the time. If you'd like to go deeper, explore techniques like diaphragmatic breathing, where you focus on fully expanding your belly with each inhale.

   When and How Often?

   Mornings can be ideal for breathwork to set a calm tone for the rest of the day. You can also practice during moments of stress, like before a challenging meeting or while sitting in traffic.

Pro tip: Pair your breathwork session with soothing music or nature sounds to enhance the relaxing effect. Apps like Calm or Headspace can guide you through the process, making it even easier to concentrate.

Limit Caffeine

High doses of caffeine can elevate cortisol and make you feel jittery. Reducing your intake can support a calmer state of mind.

- *Practical Steps*

    Gradually swap your coffee or energy drinks with substitutes like herbal teas. A few great options include:

    - *Chamomile tea*: Known for its calming properties.
    - *Rooibos tea*: Packed with antioxidants that help support stress reduction.
    - *Peppermint tea*: Naturally caffeine-free and refreshing.

If cutting coffee feels overwhelming, start small by mixing regular coffee with decaf in a 50/50 ratio or reducing to just one small cup early in the morning.

Over time, your body will adjust and rely less on caffeine for energy.

Pro tip: Add cinnamon or cardamom to herbal teas for extra flavor and an antioxidant boost!

2. ***Create an Evening Routine***: Designing a relaxing evening routine is key to improving sleep quality and reducing nighttime cortisol spikes. Your body thrives on consistency, and winding down before bed allows it to transition smoothly into restorative sleep.

Ideas to Implement

- Turn off screens at least one hour before bed. The blue light from phones, TVs, and laptops disrupts melatonin production.
- Dim the lights in your home and use warm-colored bulbs or candles to create a soothing environment.
- Engage in calming activities like reading a book, journaling, or practicing gentle stretches.
- For an extra dose of relaxation, enjoy a warm shower or bath before bed. The drop in body temperature afterward mimics natural sleep signals.

Pro tip: Add a few drops of lavender essential oil to your bath or diffuse it in your bedroom. Lavender's aroma has been shown to lower your heart rate and aid relaxation.

Days 3 & 4

1. ***Add Gentle Movement***: Gentle, restorative exercise helps lower stress hormones and soothes your nervous system without overexerting your body. Unlike intense workouts, which can temporarily spike cortisol, practices like stretching and yoga nurture calmness.

    Beginner-Friendly Routine: Dedicate 15–20 minutes to light exercise that feels enjoyable. Some great options include:

    - ***Stretching***: Try simple moves like the seated forward fold, neck rolls, or butterfly stretch.
    - ***Yoga***: Poses such as child's pose, downward dog, and cat-cow are perfect for releasing tension.
    - ***Tai Chi or Qi Gong***: These traditional practices focus on slow, graceful movements and can have a meditative effect.

    Pro tip: Look for beginner yoga videos that focus on relaxation or stretching. If you prefer to exercise outdoors, take advantage of good weather and do your stretches in a park or garden.

2. ***Mindful Walks***: Walking mindfully combines the benefits of movement with the calming power of nature. Spending time outdoors helps lower blood pressure and reduces cortisol levels.

   How to Do It

   - Head outside for a 15–20-minute walk. Leave your phone behind or keep it on silent to minimize distractions. Focus on the present moment:
   - Notice the colors around you.
   - Listen to natural sounds like birdsong or rustling leaves.
   - Feel the texture of the path under your feet, whether it's gravel, grass, or pavement.

   Pro tip: Urban dwellers can find small patches of greenery, like parks or tree-lined streets, to replicate the calming effects of nature. Even brief exposure to green spaces can dramatically improve mood.

Days 5 & 6

1. ***Cut Out Stress Triggers***: Stress isn't always about the big things; sometimes, it's the small, everyday annoyances that pile up. Identifying and minimizing these triggers can go a long way in reducing cortisol.

2. ***Take Action***: Spend a few minutes evaluating your daily routine. Write down tasks or habits that add unnecessary stress. Ask yourself:
   - Can any tasks be postponed or delegated?
   - Are social media or news apps contributing to anxiety?
   - Is your schedule leaving little room for rest or downtime?

   Once you identify these triggers, take small, intentional steps to minimize them. For example, silence non-urgent notifications or set boundaries for work-related emails after hours.

   Pro tip: Use the Eisenhower Matrix to organize tasks into four categories (urgent/important, not-urgent/important, urgent/not-important, not-urgent/not-important). This makes it easier to prioritize and cut out what isn't necessary.

3. ***Introduce Meditation***: Meditation is a proven method to lower cortisol and bring your mind into a calmer state. It helps train your brain to focus, reducing the feeling of being overwhelmed.

   <u>How to Get Started</u>
   - Sit or lie comfortably in a quiet space.
   - Close your eyes and take a few deep breaths.

- Simply focus on your breath. When your mind wanders, gently bring it back.

Guided meditations can provide structure and make the practice feel approachable. Apps like Insight Timer or YouTube channels offer options tailored for beginners.

Pro tip: Even 2–3 minutes can make a difference when done regularly. Experiment with different times of day to see what works best for you.

Day 7

Self-Care Day: Dedicate this day to nurturing your joy and well-being. Self-care isn't selfish; it's essential to reset your energy and show kindness to yourself.

Ideas for Self-Care

- Take a day off from obligations (if possible) to focus on things that make you happy.
- Spend time on a relaxing hobby like painting, knitting, or baking.
- Call a loved one and enjoy a heartfelt conversation.
- Treat yourself to a nurturing activity, like soaking in a warm bath or indulging in a good book.

Pro tip: When scheduling your week, pencil in self-care time just like any other commitment. Protect this time intentionally.

By the end of this week, take note of the progress you've made. Are you sleeping better? Do you feel calmer throughout the day? Even small improvements, like reduced tension or a more focused mind, are victories worth celebrating. You're laying the groundwork for deeper healing, and this is just the start of your cortisol reset! Be proud of the effort you've invested in your well-being.

Week 2: Nourish & Repair (Days 8–14)

Now that you've calmed your system, it's time to focus on fixing the internal damage caused by prolonged stress. This week centers on healing through nutrition and restorative practices.

Day 8-9: Fine-Tune Your Pantry and Meals

By now, you've likely made a solid start on removing processed foods and incorporating nourishing staples. These next two days are about refining and planning further to ensure consistency.

1. ***Meal Prep Time***: Dedicate an hour or two to meal prep to make healthy eating easier during busy days. Batch-cook grains (like quinoa or brown rice), roast a mix of vegetables, and prepare a large protein option (like grilled chicken, hard-boiled eggs, or lentils). Store these in containers to mix and match meals throughout the week.

Sample Prep Plan:

- Grill chicken or bake tofu cubes with olive oil and spices.
- Roast a tray of sweet potatoes, bell peppers, and zucchini.
- Wash and chop leafy greens for quick salads.
- Cook a pot of brown rice or quinoa for grain bowls.

2. ***Add Variety***: Explore food staples you haven't tried yet. For instance, swap spinach for Swiss chard or kale in a salad, or try walnuts instead of almonds as a snack. Adding variety ensures your body receives a broad range of nutrients.

Morning Energy Tip: Try starting your day with a nourishing drink like a matcha latte with almond or oat milk. Matcha contains L-theanine, which helps improve focus without causing the caffeine spikes associated with coffee.

Days 10-11: Practice Balanced Eating and Mindful Snacking

Keep building on balanced meals with some added mindfulness in how you snack and eat. Eating too quickly or skipping meals can disrupt cortisol levels, so focus on creating a relaxed rhythm with your food.

1. ***Balanced Mealtime Tips***:

- Slow down when eating. Chew your food thoroughly and put your fork down between bites. This gives your brain time to register fullness, reducing overeating and stress on your digestion.
- Don't skip meals! Skipping meals can lead to a blood sugar drop, which signals your body to release cortisol for energy.

2. ***Snack Ideas***: Prepare go-to healthy snacks ahead of time to avoid processed options.
3. ***Sweet Craving***: A small apple with a teaspoon of almond or peanut butter.
4. ***Savory Craving***: A handful of roasted chickpeas or mixed nuts.
5. ***Simple & Satisfying***: Greek yogurt with berries and a drizzle of honey.
6. ***Hydration Check***: If plain water feels repetitive, try infused water. Add cucumber, mint, or berries to your water for a refreshing twist.

Days 12-13: Introduce Adaptogens Gradually

Adaptogens are potent allies during Week 2, but they're best introduced slowly to understand how your body responds.

1. ***Easy Start***: Begin by trying one adaptogen. For instance:

- *Ashwagandha*: Start with ½ teaspoon mixed into warm milk with cinnamon, or add it to a smoothie.
    - *Tulsi Tea*: Enjoy a cup of holy basil (tulsi) tea in the afternoon to encourage a sense of calm and focus.
2. **_Trial and Error_**: Everyone's body reacts differently, so go slowly and take note of how you feel. You may find that Ashwagandha helps you sleep better, or maybe Tulsi helps you stay focused.
3. **_Daily Integration_**: Add adaptogens to foods you enjoy. For example, stir a pinch of reishi mushroom powder into your soup or blend it into your morning green smoothie.
4. **_Combine with Rituals_**: Pair adaptogens with one of your existing Week 1 rituals, like sipping reishi tea during your evening wind-down routine. This layering of habits can promote consistency and relaxation.

Day 14: Reflections and Long-Term Adaptation

Day 14 marks the end of Week 2, and it's a great time to reflect on the changes you've made to your eating habits and how they impact your stress levels.

- *Assess Your Energy*: Ask yourself how your body feels after a week of nourishing meals and cortisol-friendly foods. Do you feel a steadier energy throughout the day? Is your digestion better?

- *Favorite Recipes*: Make a list of meals and snacks that worked well for you. This will help streamline planning and ensure you stick with what you enjoy.
- *Plan for Adaptogens*: Consider which adaptogens you want to keep in your routine. For instance, you might decide to stick with Ashwagandha for stress or Tulsi tea for focus. Add these to your weekly shopping list so they're always on hand.
- *Celebrate Your Progress*: Find a simple way to acknowledge your efforts. This could be treating yourself to a cozy evening with a favorite book or preparing your favorite healthy dessert. Small rewards can motivate you to keep going.

By the end of Week 2, your body should feel stronger and more nourished. The focus on balanced meals and blood sugar stability will help reduce cortisol spikes, while adaptogens can provide extra support for handling stress. With these foundational habits in place, you're ready to transition seamlessly into Week 3, where you'll work on long-term strengthening and resilience!

Week 3: Sustain & Strengthen (Days 15–21)

Now that you have established a strong foundation of healthy eating habits and stress management techniques, Week 3 will focus on sustaining and strengthening your body's overall wellness. This week's theme is all about long-term health and building resilience to handle whatever challenges may come your way.

Day 15-16: Add Strength Training to Your Routine

Strength training doesn't have to mean heavy weights or intense gym sessions. The goal here is to incorporate light to moderate resistance exercises to boost your mood, regulate blood sugar levels, and lower cortisol.

Getting Started: Start small. Bodyweight exercises or resistance bands are enough to make a difference.

Simple Circuit: Try this beginner routine:

- 10 squats
- 8 push-ups (do them on your knees if needed)
- 30-second plank
- Repeat 2–3 rounds, pausing to rest as needed.

Stretch Afterward: Dedicate a few minutes to post-workout stretching. Moves like a seated forward fold or cat-cow pose can relieve any tension and reduce stress.

Recovery: Follow your workout with a light snack that includes protein to support muscle repair. A boiled egg with avocado slices or a handful of nuts and seeds works well.

Day 17-18: Hone Your Daily Stress-Relief Practices

You've tried several calming techniques by now. These days are about identifying what has made the biggest impact and refining those practices.

1. *Find Your Favorites*: Think about the rituals you've tried, whether it's meditation, journaling, or breathing exercises. Choose 1–2 that you've enjoyed or felt the most benefit from and make them a priority.
2. *Expand Your Practice*:
    - If mindfulness was helpful, try adding visualization. Close your eyes and imagine yourself in a peaceful, safe place, like hiking through the woods or sitting by the ocean. This can amplify relaxation.
    - If journaling made a difference, consider using prompts. Write about what triggers stress for you and, more importantly, what helps you feel grounded.
3. *Natural Support*: Sneak in time outdoors when possible. Even 15 minutes of fresh air and natural light can calm your mind and lower cortisol.

Day 19-20: Double Down on Connection and Gratitude

Cortisol levels can rise with feelings of loneliness or isolation, so these days, focus on the support and energy you can gain from people around you. Building meaningful connections can do wonders for your sense of balance.

- ***Reach Out***: Plan time with someone who lifts your spirits. This could be coffee with a friend, a family dinner, or even a phone call with someone you trust.
- ***Quality Over Quantity***: Focus on deeper, more meaningful interactions versus surface-level exchanges. Afterward, reflect on how those moments made you feel.
- ***Gratitude Practice***: Before bed, take a few minutes to write down or think about three things you're thankful for. It could be something small, like a sunny day, or something big, like support from a loved one. Shifting your mindset toward positivity can have a real impact on stress levels.

Day 21: Reflect, Reassess, and Plan for the Future

The last day of the 3-Week Cortisol Reset Plan is about looking back at what you've learned and thinking ahead. Use this time to take stock of your progress and create a sustainable routine.

1. ***Ask Yourself***: Spend some time reflecting on how far you've come.
    - Do you feel better equipped to handle stress?
    - Are your energy and mood more stable?
    - What has worked well in your routine, and what didn't feel right for you?
2. ***Set Your Intentions***: Think about the habits and rituals you want to carry forward. For example:

- Commit to strength training twice a week.
- Keep a favorite adaptogen, like Ashwagandha, part of your routine.
- Aim for at least 5 minutes of mindfulness or breathing exercises each day.

3. **Celebrate Your Progress**: Recognize the effort you've put in. Treat yourself with something that feels rewarding but also supports your well-being. Maybe it's a cozy evening with your favorite movie, trying a new healthy recipe, or indulging in a relaxing bath.

Consistency builds stronger habits and a calmer mind. Stress takes time to manage, but tools like meal prep, adaptogens, and mindfulness can help. Stay flexible, adjust as needed, and focus on progress one step at a time.

Daily Rituals for Stress Support

These simple, accessible habits can be integrated into any schedule to support cortisol balance long-term.

1. **Morning Sunlight**: Start your day right by getting at least 10–15 minutes of natural sunlight exposure within an hour of waking up. Sunlight helps regulate your circadian rhythm, boosting your mood and energy levels for the day ahead. Try stepping outside with your morning coffee or tea for some fresh air and light.
2. **Midday Stretch Break**: Take a five-minute stretching break during your workday to release built-up tension

in your muscles and reset your focus. Stretch your neck, shoulders, back, and legs to improve circulation and reduce stiffness, especially if you've been sitting for long periods.
3. ***Tech-Free Hour***: Dedicate one hour each day to unplugging from all screens—no phones, laptops, or TVs. Use this time to read a book, journal your thoughts, engage in a creative activity, or spend quality time with loved ones. This break can help you recharge mentally and improve your overall well-being.
4. ***Balanced Snacks***: Keep healthy snacks like mixed nuts, fresh fruit, or veggies with hummus on hand to maintain steady energy throughout the day. These nutrient-rich options help you avoid unhealthy cravings or energy crashes caused by processed snacks or sugary treats.
5. ***Breathing Exercises***: When stress creeps in, try diaphragmatic breathing to calm your mind and body. Take five slow, deep breaths, inhaling through your nose for a count of four, holding for a moment, and then exhaling through your mouth for a count of six. It's a quick and effective way to regain control and reduce anxiety.
6. ***Gratitude Journaling***: Before bed, write down at least one positive thing that happened during your day, no matter how small it may seem. It could be a kind gesture, a good conversation, or simply enjoying your

favorite meal. Focusing on the positives can improve your mood and help you end the day on a high note.

The 3-Week Cortisol Reset Plan equips you with tools to reclaim balance and vitality. Whether it's nourishing your body with whole foods, strengthening it with mindful movement, or calming your mind through stress-relief practices, each small step builds toward a healthier, more resilient you. Stick with what feels right for you, and remember that progress, not perfection, is the ultimate goal.

Meal Plans & Recipes

The right foods can nourish your body, regulate hormones, and support a calm mind. This chapter provides a practical guide to meals and snacks designed to balance cortisol levels. Whether you're new to healthy eating or looking for fresh ideas, these recipes are simple, satisfying, and easy to follow.

7-Day Sample Meal Plan

Here's a full week of meals to help you build routines that nurture your body and stabilize cortisol. Each day includes easy-to-prepare options for breakfast, lunch, dinner, and snacks. Adjust portion sizes based on your hunger and lifestyle.

Day 1

Breakfast: Oatmeal with chia seeds, almond butter, and fresh berries.

Snack: Handful of walnuts and a sliced apple.

Lunch: Quinoa salad with spinach, roasted sweet potatoes, grilled chicken, and tahini dressing.

Snack: Carrot sticks with hummus.

Dinner: Baked salmon with steamed broccoli and wild rice.

Day 2

Breakfast: Green smoothie with spinach, banana, almond milk, and a scoop of protein powder.

Snack: A boiled egg with cucumber slices.

Lunch: Mediterranean wrap with whole-grain tortilla, hummus, cucumber, cherry tomatoes, feta, and olives.

Snack: Handful of mixed nuts.

Dinner: Stir-fry with tofu, zucchini, mushrooms, and brown rice.

Day 3

Breakfast: Overnight oats with cinnamon, flaxseeds, and a dollop of Greek yogurt.

Snack: Orange segments with a sprinkle of almonds.

Lunch: Lentil soup with a side of mixed greens and olive oil dressing.

Snack: Sliced avocado with lemon and sea salt.

Dinner: Grilled chicken with mashed sweet potatoes and sautéed asparagus.

Day 4

Breakfast: Veggie scramble (eggs, spinach, mushrooms) with a slice of whole-grain toast.

Snack: A handful of roasted chickpeas.

Lunch: Grain bowl with farro, roasted vegetables, and tahini dressing.

Snack: Sliced carrots and bell peppers with guacamole.

Dinner: Herbal roasted turkey breast with steamed Brussels sprouts and quinoa.

Day 5

Breakfast: Smoothie bowl with frozen mixed berries, almond milk, and chia seeds, topped with granola.

Snack: A banana with almond butter.

Lunch: Arugula salad with grilled shrimp, avocado slices, and a lemon vinaigrette.

Snack: Few squares of dark chocolate with a handful of pistachios.

Dinner: Ginger-turmeric cod with roasted sweet potatoes and sautéed kale.

Day 6

Breakfast: Greek yogurt parfait layered with granola, blueberries, and chia seeds.

Snack: Sliced pear with a small handful of walnuts.

Lunch: Lentil and veggie-stuffed bell peppers.

Snack: Roasted almonds and a piece of dark chocolate.

Dinner: Seared chicken thighs with steamed broccoli and brown rice pilaf.

Day 7

Breakfast: Avocado toast on whole-grain bread with a poached egg.

Snack: A fruit smoothie with spinach, frozen mango, and a scoop of protein powder.

Lunch: Buddha bowl with quinoa, roasted veggies, chickpeas, and a tahini drizzle.

Snack: Handful of trail mix (nuts, seeds, dried fruit).

Dinner: Baked salmon with roasted carrots and sautéed spinach.

Cortisol-Balancing Breakfasts

Mornings set the tone for your day, so fueling your body with nutrient-dense, cortisol-friendly foods is key. Below are a few simple, delicious breakfast recipes to kickstart your day.

Overnight Chia Oats

Ingredients:

- 1/2 cup rolled oats
- 1 tablespoon chia seeds
- 1 cup almond milk (or milk of your choice)
- 1/2 teaspoon cinnamon
- 1/4 cup fresh berries

Instructions:

1. Combine oats, chia seeds, almond milk, and cinnamon in a jar or container with a lid.
2. Stir well, cover, and refrigerate overnight.
3. Top with fresh berries in the morning and enjoy cold or warmed up.

Veggie Breakfast Scramble

Ingredients:

- 2 eggs
- 1/4 cup chopped spinach
- 1/4 cup diced mushrooms
- 1/4 cup diced red bell peppers
- 1 teaspoon olive oil

Instructions:

1. Heat olive oil in a skillet over medium heat.
2. Sauté mushrooms, peppers, and spinach for 2–3 minutes.
3. Crack eggs into the skillet and scramble until fully cooked.

Protein-Packed Smoothie Bowl

Ingredients:

- 1/2 frozen banana
- 1/2 cup frozen mixed berries
- 1 tablespoon almond butter
- 1 scoop protein powder
- 3/4 cup almond milk

Instructions:

1. In a blender, combine frozen banana, mixed berries, almond butter, protein powder, and almond milk.
2. Blend until smooth and creamy.
3. Pour into a bowl and top with your choice of toppings such as granola, chia seeds, or fresh fruit.

Energy-Stabilizing Lunches

Midday meals are critical for keeping your energy levels consistent throughout the day. These recipes focus on balanced macronutrients to keep you energized and stress-free.

Quinoa Salad with Roasted Vegetables

Ingredients:

- 1 cup cooked quinoa
- 1/2 cup roasted sweet potatoes
- 1/4 cup roasted zucchini
- 1/4 cup chopped spinach
- 2 tablespoons tahini dressing

Instructions:

1. Toss all ingredients in a large bowl.
2. Drizzle with tahini dressing and serve.

Lentil and Arugula Salad

Ingredients:

- 1/2 cup cooked lentils
- 2 cups arugula
- 1/4 cup cherry tomatoes (halved)
- 1 tablespoon olive oil
- Squeeze of fresh lemon juice

Instructions:

1. Combine lentils, arugula, and tomatoes in a bowl.
2. Drizzle with olive oil and lemon juice, tossing to coat.

Mediterranean Veggie Wrap

Ingredients:

- 1 whole-grain wrap
- 2 tablespoons hummus
- 1/4 cup diced cucumbers
- 1/4 cup cherry tomatoes (diced)
- 1 tablespoon crumbled feta cheese

Instructions:

1. Spread hummus over the wrap.
2. Layer with cucumbers, tomatoes, and feta. Roll tightly and slice in half.

Hormone-Supportive Dinners

Salmon and Broccoli Dinner

Ingredients:

- 1 salmon fillet
- 1 cup steamed broccoli
- 1/2 cup cooked wild rice
- 1 teaspoon olive oil

Instructions:

1. Bake salmon at 375°F for 12–15 minutes.
2. Serve with steamed broccoli and wild rice, drizzling olive oil over everything.

Chicken Stir-Fry with Veggies

Ingredients:

- 1 cup cooked brown rice
- 1 chicken breast (sliced)
- 1/4 cup sliced zucchini
- 1/4 cup sliced mushrooms
- 1 tablespoon low-sodium soy sauce

Instructions:

1. Sauté chicken until fully cooked, then set aside.
2. Stir-fry vegetables in the same pan for 5 minutes.
3. Add chicken back in and mix with soy sauce. Serve over rice.

Turmeric Cod with Sweet Potatoes

Ingredients:

- 1 cod fillet
- 1/2 teaspoon turmeric powder
- 1 medium sweet potato (baked)

Instructions:

1. Rub turmeric on the cod fillet and bake at 375°F for 15 minutes.
2. Serve with the baked sweet potato and garnish with parsley.

Calming Teas, Snacks & Smoothies

Introducing calming teas, snacks, and smoothies into your routine is a simple yet effective way to promote relaxation, stabilize energy levels, and support your body's stress response. These recipes are designed to be easy to prepare and packed with cortisol-friendly ingredients that help balance your hormones and nourish your mind and body.

Calming Teas

Chamomile Lavender Tea

Ingredients:

- 1 chamomile tea bag or 1 tablespoon dried chamomile flowers
- 1/2 teaspoon dried lavender
- 1 cup hot water
- 1 teaspoon raw honey (optional)

Instructions:

1. Add the chamomile and lavender to a teapot or mug.
2. Pour hot water over the herbs and steep for 5–7 minutes.
3. Strain or remove the tea bag, and stir in honey if desired. Sip slowly before bed for a restful night.

Ginger-Turmeric Tea

Ingredients:

- 1-inch piece of fresh ginger (sliced)
- 1/2 teaspoon ground turmeric or 1 teaspoon fresh turmeric (grated)
- 1 cup hot water
- Lemon slices and honey for flavor (optional)

Instructions:

1. Add ginger and turmeric to a pot of hot water. Simmer for 10 minutes.
2. Strain into a mug and squeeze in lemon juice. Add honey to sweeten, if desired.

Holy Basil (Tulsi) Tea

Ingredients:

- 1 tablespoon dried holy basil leaves or 1 tea bag
- 1 cup hot water
- 1 teaspoon coconut sugar or raw honey (optional)

Instructions:

1. Brew holy basil tea by steeping the leaves or tea bag in hot water for 5–7 minutes.
2. Sweeten with honey or coconut sugar as desired. Enjoy during a mid-afternoon break for a calming pause.

Nutrient-Dense Snacks

Coconut Chia Seed Energy Bites

Ingredients:

- 1/2 cup almond butter
- 1/4 cup shredded coconut
- 2 tablespoons chia seeds
- 2 tablespoons honey
- 1/2 cup rolled oats

Instructions:

1. Mix all ingredients in a bowl until well combined.
2. Roll into small balls (about 1 inch in diameter).
3. Refrigerate for 30 minutes to firm up. Keep stored in an airtight container for up to one week.

Roasted Chickpeas with Spices

Ingredients:

- 1 can (15 oz) chickpeas, drained and rinsed
- 1 tablespoon olive oil
- 1 teaspoon smoked paprika
- 1/2 teaspoon garlic powder
- 1/4 teaspoon sea salt

Instructions:

1. Preheat oven to 400°F (200°C).
2. Toss chickpeas with olive oil and spices until evenly coated.
3. Spread on a baking sheet in a single layer.
4. Roast for 25–30 minutes, shaking the pan halfway through, until crispy.

Sliced Veggies with Avocado Dip

Ingredients:

- 1 ripe avocado
- Juice of 1 lime
- Pinch of sea salt
- Veggie sticks (carrots, celery, and cucumber)

Instructions:

1. Mash the avocado with lime juice and salt until smooth.
2. Serve with sliced veggie sticks for dipping.

Relaxing Smoothies

Blueberry-Banana Calm Smoothie

Ingredients:

- 1/2 frozen banana
- 1/2 cup fresh or frozen blueberries
- 1/2 cup unsweetened almond milk
- 1 tablespoon flaxseeds
- 1 teaspoon raw honey (optional)

Instructions:

1. Blend all ingredients until smooth.
2. Pour into a glass and enjoy as a mid-morning or afternoon snack.

Ashwagandha Adaptogen Smoothie

Ingredients:

- 1 cup spinach
- 1/2 frozen banana
- 1/4 cup frozen mango
- 1/2 teaspoon ashwagandha powder
- 1 cup coconut water

Instructions:

1. Add all ingredients to a blender and blend until creamy.
2. Serve immediately and enjoy the calming effects.

Chocolate Almond Bliss Smoothie

Ingredients:

- 1 cup unsweetened almond milk
- 1 tablespoon almond butter
- 1 tablespoon raw cacao powder
- 1/2 frozen banana
- 1/2 cup ice

Instructions:

1. Combine all ingredients in a blender and blend until smooth.
2. Pour into a glass and enjoy as a stress-relieving treat.

By incorporating these teas, snacks, and smoothies into your day, you can create pockets of calm that help balance cortisol and support your body's relaxation response. Treat these as moments of self-care and enjoy the benefits of nourishing yourself from the inside out.

Lifestyle Habits That Reset Cortisol

Managing stress and balancing cortisol levels isn't just about what you eat or drink. Your daily habits and routines play an equally important role. Simple adjustments to your lifestyle can make a profound difference in how you feel, equipping your body and mind to better handle stress. This chapter will walk you through practical steps for incorporating gentle movement, improving sleep, practicing calming techniques, and minimizing external stress triggers.

Gentle Movement & Walking Protocols

Exercise can either support or hinder cortisol balance, depending on intensity and duration. While intense workouts may lead to temporary cortisol spikes, gentle movement helps to reduce stress hormones and encourage relaxation.

Why Gentle Movement Works

Low-impact activities keep your body energized without overwhelming your nervous system. Practices like walking, yoga, or tai chi can lower cortisol levels, improve circulation, and clear your mind.

Walking Protocol for Cortisol Balance

Walking is one of the easiest and most effective movements to incorporate into your day. It requires no equipment and can fit into even the busiest schedules.

- *Duration*: Walk for 20–30 minutes daily.
- *Setting*: Choose calm environments, like parks, trails, or quiet neighborhoods. If you're stuck indoors, use a treadmill at a leisurely pace.
- *Mindful Walking*: Leave headphones at home and focus on the rhythm of your steps, the sound of birds, or the feel of fresh air on your skin. This mindful approach enhances relaxation.

Yoga for Beginners

Yoga combines movement and deep breathing, making it particularly effective in managing cortisol. Here's how to get started:

- *Start Small*: Attend a gentle or restorative yoga class or follow a beginner-friendly online video at home.
- *Routine Poses*: Try easy poses like Child's Pose (Balasana), Cat-Cow Pose, and Legs-Up-the-Wall Pose, which are known for their calming effects.

Pro Tip: Schedule your walks or yoga sessions during your most stressful times of day, such as early morning or post-work, to help regulate cortisol rhythms.

Sleep Optimization

Cortisol and sleep are deeply interconnected. Poor sleep quality or insufficient rest can cause your cortisol levels to remain elevated, while solid, restorative sleep can bring them back into balance.

Crafting a Bedtime Routine

Your body thrives on consistency, so creating a calming evening routine can prepare your brain for sleep.

1. *Wind Down Early*: Start your bedtime routine 30–60 minutes before sleep.
2. *Limit Stimulants*: Avoid caffeine after mid-afternoon and skip large meals or alcohol before bed.
3. *Relaxing Activities*: Engage in calming rituals like reading a book, stretching, or listening to soothing music.

Optimize Your Sleep Environment

Your bedroom setup can make or break your sleep quality. Here's how to create the perfect space for restful nights:

- *Dim Lighting*: Use soft, warm lights in the evening, and consider blackout curtains or an eye mask to block out light.
- *Comfortable Temperature*: Keep your room cool, ideally between 60–67°F (15–19°C).
- *Declutter*: A tidy and minimal bedroom can promote calmness and reduce stress.

Managing Nighttime Stress

Sometimes, a racing mind keeps you from falling asleep. Address this by jotting down worries in a notebook or doing a short meditation session before bed. Apps with guided meditations or sleep stories can also help quiet an anxious mind.

Pro Tip: Aim for 7–9 hours of sleep each night, and try to go to bed and wake up at the same time daily to establish consistent circadian rhythms.

Breathing Exercises & Grounding Techniques

Your breath is one of the most powerful (and free!) tools you have to calm the nervous system and lower cortisol levels. Grounding techniques further help to shift your focus away from stress by reconnecting you to the present moment.

Breathing Exercises

Practicing conscious breathing can activate your parasympathetic nervous system, signaling your body to relax.

1. *4-7-8 Breathing Method*

This technique slows your breathing and lowers cortisol in minutes.

Instructions:

- Exhale completely through your mouth.
- Inhale quietly through your nose for a count of 4.
- Hold your breath for a count of 7.
- Exhale audibly through your mouth for a count of 8.
- Repeat the cycle 4 times.

2. *Box Breathing*

Ideal for high-stress moments, this method brings your focus to your breath.

Instructions:

- Breathe in through your nose for a count of 4.
- Hold your breath for a count of 4.
- Exhale through your mouth for a count of 4.
- Hold your breath again for a count of 4.

- Repeat for 1–2 minutes.

Grounding Techniques

Grounding exercises bring you back to the present, helping to break the cycle of overthinking.

1. *5-4-3-2-1 Technique*

   This simple mindfulness exercise uses your senses to center your mind.

   - Identify 5 things you can see around you.
   - Identify 4 things you can physically feel.
   - Identify 3 things you can hear.
   - Identify 2 things you can smell.
   - Identify 1 thing you can taste.

2. *Earthing*

   Reconnect with nature by walking barefoot on grass, sand, or dirt. The physical contact with the earth's surface has been shown to reduce cortisol and inflammation.

   Pro Tip: Dedicate 5–10 minutes daily to breathing or grounding exercises. Over time, you'll notice their cumulative calming effects.

Reducing Screen Time and Cortisol Triggers

Today's digital world is filled with constant notifications, emails, and social media updates that keep your cortisol on overdrive. Cutting back on screen time and avoiding common triggers can have a profound impact on your stress levels.

Why Screen Time Affects Cortisol

Excessive exposure to screens, especially in the evening, disrupts your natural cortisol rhythm and melatonin production. Blue light from screens tricks your brain into thinking it's daytime, making it harder to wind down.

Strategies to Reduce Screen Time

1. *Establish "Digital Curfews"*: Turn off devices at least 1 hour before bedtime. Use this time for relaxing activities like reading or journaling.
2. *Limit Notifications*: Disable non-essential phone notifications to prevent constant interruptions during the day.
3. *Batch Social Media Time*: Instead of checking social media throughout the day, dedicate specific 10–15 minute blocks to scrolling and stick to them.

Avoiding Cortisol Triggers

Certain habits and activities can spike cortisol unnecessarily. Here's how to identify and reduce them:

- ***Late-Night Emails***: If possible, avoid checking work emails after hours to protect your evening wind-down time. Set boundaries for when you're online and offline.
- ***Stressing News Cycles***: A constant influx of negative news can raise your stress levels. Consider limiting your news consumption to one check-in per day.
- ***Overcommitting***: Learn to say no to excessive obligations. Prioritize activities that align with your health and well-being goals.

Pro Tip: Use apps like "Screen Time" or "Digital Wellbeing" to monitor your device usage and keep it in check.

Reset your cortisol levels by building sustainable habits like gentle movement, better sleep, calming techniques, and less screen time. These small changes promote balance, resilience, and control over stress.

Beyond the Reset: Long-Term Stress Management

Managing stress is an ongoing process that requires continuous effort and mindful awareness. While a reset can provide immediate relief, it's important to continue implementing healthy habits in your daily routine to maintain balanced cortisol levels and overall well-being.

How to Reintroduce Foods Without Relapse

During the reset, you may have excluded certain foods to help regulate cortisol and reduce stress on your body. Now, it's time to reintroduce those foods gradually to test how your body responds while maintaining the balance you've worked hard to achieve.

1. **Go Slowly**

    Reintroducing foods too quickly can overwhelm your body and make it difficult to pinpoint any foods that may be problematic. Follow these steps to avoid a relapse:

- Introduce one food at a time, waiting 3–5 days before adding the next food. This allows you to observe how your body reacts.
- Start with small portions, then gradually increase over the following days if your body tolerates it well.

2. **Watch for Triggers**

Some foods can cause inflammation, bloating, fatigue, or even heightened stress levels. Below are signs to look for:

- ***Physical Symptoms***: Digestive issues, headaches, acne, or joint pain.
- ***Mental Symptoms***: Trouble sleeping, feeling anxious, or increased irritability.

3. **Balance Is Key**

Even as you reintroduce foods, focus on maintaining a nutrient-dense diet with plenty of whole foods, fiber, healthy fats, and lean proteins. Treat indulgent foods like sweets or alcohol as occasional treats rather than daily staples.

Example Approach:

- *Week 1*: Reintroduce dairy. Try a serving of Greek yogurt or cheese and monitor for 3–5 days.

- **Week 2**: Reintroduce gluten. Test bread or pasta and track your body's response.
- **Week 3**: Reintroduce moderately processed foods, such as crackers or store-bought dressings.

<u>**Pro Tip**</u>: Keep a food journal to track what you eat and how you feel. This will help you identify patterns and potential sensitivities.

Building Resilience: Mental & Physical

Achieving long-term cortisol balance means strengthening your mind and body to handle life's unavoidable stressors. Resilience allows you to recover from challenges with greater ease and confidence.

1. <u>**Strengthen Your Mind**</u>: Cultivating mental resilience can help you approach stress with a sense of calm and control.
   - *Practice Mindfulness*: Spend 5–10 minutes daily meditating or focusing on your breath. Use apps like Headspace or Calm for guided meditations.
   - *Daily Gratitude*: Start each day by writing down three things you're grateful for. This rewires your brain to focus on positivity and lowers stress over time.

- ○ ***Build Healthy Relationships***: Surround yourself with supportive people who uplift and inspire you. Strong social connections act as a buffer against stress.
2. **Nourish Your Body**: Physical resilience comes from consistently caring for your body through movement, rest, and nourishment.
    - ○ ***Regular Movement***: Include a mix of strength training, cardio, and activities like yoga or hikes. Aim for at least 150 minutes of moderate exercise per week.
    - ○ ***Stay Hydrated***: Dehydration can increase cortisol levels, so drink at least 8–10 glasses of water daily. Add a splash of lemon or cucumber for a refreshing twist.
    - ○ ***Eat Nutrient-Dense Meals***: Focus on whole foods with plenty of antioxidants, healthy fats, and protein to support hormonal balance.
3. **Prioritize Recovery**: Resilience isn't about always being on the go. Rest and recovery are just as important:
    - ○ Schedule rest days in your workout routine.
    - ○ Include restorative practices like stretching, foam rolling, or using a sauna.

Pro Tip: Challenge yourself with small hurdles like learning a new skill, which builds mental toughness and confidence over time.

Monitoring Progress and Listening to Your Body

Cortisol balance is not static; it requires ongoing awareness and adjustments. Monitoring progress helps you stay aligned with your health goals and catch imbalances early.

1. **Track Your Progress**

    Regularly checking in with your body ensures that you stay on the right track.

    Journaling: Keep a notebook to record your energy levels, mood, sleep quality, and any physical symptoms. Use prompts like:

    - "What energized me today?"
    - "How did I handle stress today?"

    Apps to Try: Apps like MyFitnessPal for tracking meals, or mood-tracking apps like Daylio, can simplify the process.

2. **Recognize Imbalances**

    Life happens, and stress can creep back in. Here are some warning signs of cortisol imbalance to look out for:

    - Difficulty sleeping or waking up exhausted.
    - Increased cravings for sugar or caffeine.

- Feeling anxious, overwhelmed, or irritable frequently.
- Gaining or losing weight unexpectedly.

3. **Adjust Habits as Needed**

   When you notice something feels "off," tweak your habits instead of waiting for the issue to worsen.

   - If sleep suffers, revisit your bedtime routine.
   - If fatigue is a problem, ensure you're eating enough and consider incorporating adaptogens like ashwagandha.
   - If stress feels overwhelming, revisit grounding techniques or mindfulness practices.

Pro Tip: Reflect monthly on your progress by asking, "What's working?" and "What needs to change?"

When to Seek Help: Doctors, Labs, & Next Steps

Despite your best efforts, you may need professional guidance to fully address chronic stress or cortisol imbalances. Seeking help is a proactive step toward better health.

1. **When to Consult a Doctor:**

   Consider consulting a healthcare professional if you experience the following:

- Prolonged fatigue or difficulty getting out of bed despite adequate sleep.
- Persistent anxiety, irritability, or brain fog.
- Unexplained weight gain, particularly around the midsection.
- Regular illness or slow recovery from colds and infections.

2. **What Tests to Request:**

A few lab tests can provide a better picture of your cortisol levels and overall health:

- ***Salivary Cortisol Test***: Measures cortisol levels throughout the day to identify imbalances.
- ***Comprehensive Hormone Panel***: Assesses levels of other hormones like DHEA, estrogen, and testosterone.
- ***Thyroid Panel***: Thyroid health impacts cortisol, so checking TSH, T3, and T4 is valuable.
- ***Nutrient Deficiency Tests***: Identify deficiencies in magnesium, vitamin D, or B vitamins, which can impact stress and energy.

3. **Working with Your Doctor:**

Be clear and assertive about your concerns when speaking with your doctor. Share detailed notes about your symptoms and lifestyle changes. Ask for advice tailored to your situation.

4. **Next Steps for Ongoing Support:**

   Consider working with other specialists if needed, such as:

   - ***Functional Medicine Practitioners***: They focus on holistic and personalized approaches, often addressing root causes of stress.
   - ***Registered Dietitians***: Helpful for creating meal plans to further support hormonal balance.
   - ***Therapists***: Cognitive-behavioral therapy (CBT) or mindfulness-based therapy can help manage stress mentally.

Balancing cortisol long-term is about building small, consistent habits to support your health. Gradually reintroduce foods, build resilience, listen to your body, and seek help when needed to maintain balance and reduce stress. Use this phase to better understand your body's needs.

Conclusion

By reaching the end of this guide, you've already taken a monumental step toward better understanding your health and the role of cortisol in your life. This isn't just about stress management; it's about creating a life that feels balanced, intentional, and vibrant.

Throughout this guide, you've explored the science of cortisol, its effects on your body, and how it uniquely impacts women's health. You've learned that small, consistent changes can be powerful—from incorporating anti-inflammatory foods into your meals, to establishing calming nighttime routines, to finding joy in mindful movement. These adjustments form the foundation for resetting your cortisol and building resilience.

The beauty of this process lies in its simplicity. You don't need to overhaul your lifestyle overnight. Instead, focus on the small choices you make each day, like taking a moment to breathe deeply, replacing one cup of coffee with herbal tea, or spending an afternoon outdoors. These micro-changes add up, creating lasting improvements in how your body handles stress.

Of course, progress won't always be linear, and some days may feel tougher than others. That's okay. Give yourself the grace to adapt and keep going. Your commitment to understanding and respecting your body's needs is a form of self-care that will only grow stronger with time.

Thank you for dedicating this space in your life to understanding your health. You deserve to feel energized, calm, and centered. Now's the time to put what you've learned into action. Start small, stay consistent, and remember that every positive step matters. You've equipped yourself with the tools to thrive, and an empowered, healthier you is well within reach.

FAQs

What is cortisol, and why is it important for women's health?

Cortisol is a hormone produced by the adrenal glands that helps regulate stress, metabolism, blood sugar levels, and sleep-wake cycles. For women, cortisol plays a key role in hormonal balance, energy levels, and overall health. When cortisol is out of balance, it can lead to fatigue, weight gain, irregular menstrual cycles, and mood swings.

How does chronic stress affect cortisol levels?

Chronic stress keeps cortisol levels elevated for long periods. This can disrupt your body's natural rhythm, leading to negative effects like trouble sleeping, increased belly fat, weakened immunity, and even hormonal imbalances. Over time, constant activation of the stress response can exhaust the adrenal glands, leading to low cortisol output and extreme fatigue.

What are some common symptoms of cortisol imbalance in women?

Symptoms of cortisol imbalance can include fatigue, cravings for sugar or salty foods, weight gain (especially around the abdomen), difficulty sleeping, mood swings, irregular periods, and digestive issues. You may also feel anxious, find it hard to concentrate, or experience constant low energy despite rest.

Does diet affect cortisol levels?

Yes, diet greatly impacts cortisol. Foods high in processed sugar and refined carbs can cause blood sugar spikes, triggering cortisol release. On the other hand, nutrient-dense, anti-inflammatory foods like leafy greens, berries, salmon, and whole grains help regulate cortisol and reduce stress-related inflammation.

Can exercise impact cortisol levels?

Exercise has a dual effect on cortisol. Intense workouts can temporarily raise cortisol, especially if done too often without recovery time. However, gentle movements like yoga, walking, and stretching can reduce cortisol and promote relaxation. It's important to find a balance that works for your body.

How do sleep and cortisol relate to each other?

Cortisol follows a daily rhythm, peaking in the morning to help you wake up and dropping at night for restful sleep. Poor sleep disrupts this cycle, keeping cortisol elevated into the evening and making it harder to fall asleep. Prioritizing good sleep habits, like having a consistent bedtime and limiting screen use at night, can help regulate cortisol.

What natural methods can help lower cortisol?

Several strategies can help reduce cortisol naturally, including deep breathing exercises, mindfulness meditation, spending time in nature, and practicing yoga. Consuming magnesium-rich foods (like spinach, nuts, and seeds), reducing caffeine intake, and incorporating adaptogens such as ashwagandha or holy basil can also support cortisol regulation.

References and Helpful Links

Cpt, K. D. M. R. (2024, January 29). 11 natural ways to lower your cortisol levels. Healthline.
https://www.healthline.com/nutrition/ways-to-lower-cortisol

Professional, C. C. M. (2025a, February 17). Cortisol. Cleveland Clinic.
https://my.clevelandclinic.org/health/articles/22187-cortisol#:~:text=low%20blood%20pressure.-,Helping%20control%20your%20sleep%2Dwake%20cycle,how%20your%20body%20wakes%20up.

Hospital, B. (2024, August 10). Understanding high cortisol levels in females. Benenden Health.
https://www.benendenhospital.org.uk/health-news/womens-health/understanding-high-cortisol-levels-in-females/

How to lower your cortisol levels. (n.d.). Henry Ford Health - Detroit, MI.
https://www.henryford.com/blog/2020/05/how-to-lower-your-cortisol-levels

Clinic, C. (2024, October 18). De-Stress eating: Foods to help reduce anxiety. Cleveland Clinic.
https://health.clevelandclinic.org/eat-these-foods-to-reduce-stress-and-anxiety

Nista, J. (2025, March 11). 7-Day meal plan for lower cortisol. Clean Eatz Kitchen.

https://www.cleaneatzkitchen.com/a/blog/7-day-meal-plan-for-lower-cort isol?srsltid=AfmBOor-3beICH-E3FuULvsDu6fvYaGAgqfH5MH28dfI8 D1GDXxFbyWE

Pedersen, J., Rasmussen, M. G. B., Sørensen, S. O., Mortensen, S. R., Olesen, L. G., Brage, S., Kristensen, P. L., Puterman, E., & Grøntved, A. (2022). Effects of limiting digital screen use on well-being, mood, and biomarkers of stress in adults. Npj Mental Health Research, 1(1). https://doi.org/10.1038/s44184-022-00015-6

www.ingramcontent.com/pod-product-compliance
Lightning Source LLC
LaVergne TN
LVHW012029060526
838201LV00061B/4526